CONTENTS

What Is the Optavia Diet?

The Optavia Diet is the brainchild of the man behind the multimillion-dollar company Medifast– Dr. William Vitale. Now carrying the brand Optavia since 2017, the goal of this diet is to encourage healthy and sustainable weight loss among its clientele. While there are many types of diet regimen that are available in the market, the Optavia Diet is ranked in the top 30 Best Diets in the United States.

Under this diet regimen, dieters are required to follow a weight plan that includes five feelings a day and one lean green meal daily. However, there are also other regimens of the Optavia Diet if the five fuelings a day is too much for you. And since this is a commercial diet, you have access to Optavia coaches and become part of a community that will encourage you to succeed in your weight loss journey. Moreover, this diet is also designed for people who want to transition from their old habits to healthier ones. Basically, this diet regimen is not only for people who want to lose weight but also for people who suffer from diabetes, people suffering from gout, nursing moms, seniors as well as teens.

The Optavia Diet has been subjected to various studies to prove its efficacy in weight loss. Different studies were published in various journals indicating that those who follow this program are able to see significant changes in as little as 8 weeks and that people can achieve their long-term health goals with the Optavia Diet.

The Benefits of The Optavia Diet

The Optavia Diet, similar to other weight loss programs, promises people a high success rate. However, unlike other programs, this particular diet regimen is not only easy to follow but it is also great for those who have long-term health goals. Thus, below are the benefits of following this diet regimen.

- **Structured Eating Plan:** The Optavia Diet has a structured eating plan thus making it one of the most no-brainer diets there is. Everything is spelled out for you so there is no need for you to figure out if you are following the diet correctly. Since it is very easy to follow, it is perfect for people who are always busy or do not have a knack for cooking their food.

- **Great for People Practicing Portion Control:** One of the most challenging parts of dieting is learning how to do portion control and sticking by it. The Optavia Diet comes with the Fueling phase that helps keep your meals in check so there is no need for you to eat unnecessarily.

- **Practice Long-Term Relationship with Food:** The guidance of the community following the Optavia Diet can help improve a positive long-term relationship with food. Over time, you become aware of the types of foods that you are allowed to eat and gain an appreciation of the healthy options that you have.

- **Does Not Need an Accountability Partner:** While some diets encourage you to have a diet buddy, the Optavia Diet is perfect for people who do not have accountability partners. The thing is that people are connected to a community of dieters that can provide the support needed while going through the phases of this diet.

- **Better Overall Health:** This particular diet regimen is known to help improve overall wellness. Aside from weight loss, various studies have also noted that the Optavia Diet can help people maintain stable blood pressure and blood sugar levels due to the limited sodium intake that the food contains. In fact, the Optavia provides less than 2,300 milligrams of Sodium daily.

A Deeper Look into The Optavia Diet

The Optavia Diet encourages people to limit the number of calories that they should take daily. Under this program, dieters are encouraged to consume between 800 and 1000 calories daily. For this to be possible, dieters are encouraged to opt for healthier food items as well as meal replacements. But unlike other types of commercial diet regimens, the Optavia Diet comes in different variations. There are currently three variations of the Optavia Diet plan that one can choose from according to one's needs.

- **5&1 Optavia Diet Plan:** This is the most common version of the Optavia Diet and it involves eating five prepackaged meals from the Optimal Health Fuelings and one home-made balanced meal.

- **4&2&1 Octavia Diet Plan:** This diet plan is designed for people who want to have flexibility while following this regimen. Under this program, dieters are encouraged to eat more calories and have more flexible food choices. This means that they can consume 4 prepackaged Optimal Health Fuelings food, three home-cooked meals from the Lean and Green, and one snack daily.

- **5&2&2 Optavia Diet Plan:** This diet plan is perfect for individuals who prefer to have a flexible meal plan in order to achieve a healthy weight. It is recommended for a wide variety of people. Under this diet regimen, dieters are required to eat 5 fuelings, 2 lean and green meals, and 2 healthy snacks.

- **3&3 Optavia Diet Plan:** This particular Diet plan is created for people who have moderate weight problems and merely want to maintain a healthy body. Under this diet plan, dieters are encouraged to consume 3 prepackaged Optimal Health Fuelings and three home-cooked meals.

- **Optavia for Nursing Mothers:** This diet regimen is designed for nursing mothers with babies of at least two months old. Aside from supporting breastfeeding mothers, it also encourages gradual weight loss.

- **Optavia for Diabetes:**This Optavia Diet plan is designed for people who have Type 1 and Type 2 diabetes. The meal plans are designed so that dieters consume more green and lean meals depending on their needs and condition.

- **Optavia for Gout:**This diet regimen incorporates a balance of foods that are low in purines and moderate in protein.

- **Optavia for Seniors (65 years and older):**Designed for seniors, this Optavia Diet plan has some variations following the components of Fuelings depending on the needs and activities of the senior dieters.

- **Optavia for Teen Boys and Optavia for Teen Girls (13-18 years old):**Designed for active teens, the Optavia for Teens Boys and Optavia for Teens Girls provide the right nutrition to growing teens.

Regardless of which type of Optavia Diet plan you choose, it is important that you talk with a coach to help you determine which plan is right for you based on your individual goals. This is to ensure that you get the most out of the plan that you have chosen.

How to Start This Diet

The Optavia Diet is comprised of different phases. A certified coach will educate you on the steps that you need to undertake if you want to follow this regimen. But for the sake of those who are new to this diet, below are some of the things that you need to know especially when you are still starting with this diet regimen.

Initial Steps

During this phase, people are encouraged to consume800 to 1,000 calories to help you shed off at least 12 pounds within the next 12 weeks. For instance, if you are following the 5&1 Optavia Diet Plan, then you need to eat 1 meal every 2 or 3 hours and include a 30-minute moderate workout most days of your week. You need to consume not more than 100 grams of Carbs daily during this phase.

Further, consuming the Lean and Green meals are highly encouraged. It involves eating 5 to 7 ounces of cooked lean proteins and three servings of non-starchy vegetables, and two servings of healthy fats. This phase also encourages the dieter to include 1 optional snack per day such as ½ cup sugar-free gelatin,3 celery sticks, and 12 ounces nuts. Aside from these things, below are other things that you need to remember when following this phase:

- Make sure that the portion size recommendations are for cooked weight and not the raw weight of your ingredients
- Opt for meals that are baked, grilled, broiled, or poached. Avoid frying foods as this will increase your calorie intake.
- Eat at least two servings of fish rich in Omega-3 fatty acids. These include fishes like tuna, salmon, trout, mackerel, herring, and other cold-water fishes.
- Choose meatless alternatives like tofu and tempeh.
- Follow the program even when you are dining out. Keep in mind that drinking alcohol is discouraged when following this plan.

Maintenance Phase

As soon as you have achieved your desired weight, the next phase is the transition stage. It is a 6-week stage that involves increasing your calorie intake to 1,550 per day. This is also the phase when you are allowed to add more varieties into your meal such as whole grains, low-fat dairy, and fruits.

After six weeks, you can now move into the 3&3 Optavia Diet plan, so you are required to eat three Lean and Green meals and 3 Fueling foods.

What CAN I Eat and NOT Eat?

There are so many foods that you can eat while following the Optavia Diet. However, you must know these foods by heart. This is especially true if you are just new to this diet and you have to strictly follow the 5&1 Optavia Diet Plan. Thus, this section is dedicated to the types of foods that you are allowed and not allowed to eat while following this diet regimen.

Foods That Are Allowed

There are several categories of foods that can be eaten under this diet regimen. This section will break down the Lean and Green foods that you can eat while following this diet regime.

The Lean Foods

Leanest Foods - These foods are considered to be the leanest as it has only up to 4 grams of total fat. Moreover, dieters should eat a 7-ounce cooked portion of these foods. Consume these foods with 1 healthy fat serving.
- **Fish:**Flounder, cod, haddock, grouper, Mahi, tilapia, tuna (yellowfin fresh or canned), and wild catfish.
- **Shellfish:**Scallops, lobster, crabs, shrimp
- **Game meat:**Elk, deer, buffalo
- **Ground turkey or other meat:**Should be 98% lean
- **Meatless alternatives:**14 egg whites, 2 cups egg substitute, 5 ounces seitan, 1 ½ cups 1% cottage cheese, and 12 ounces non-fat 0% Greek yogurt

Leaner Foods - These foods contain 5 to 9 grams of total fat. Consume these foods with 1 healthy fat serving. Make sure to consume only 6 ounces of a cooked portion of these foods daily:

- **Fish:** Halibut, trout, and swordfish
- **Chicken:** White meat such as breasts as long as the skin is removed
- **Turkey:** Ground turkey as long as it is 95% to 97% lean.
- **Meatless options:** 2 whole eggs plus 4 egg whites, 2 whole eggs plus one cup egg substitute, 1 ½ cups 2% cottage cheese, and 12 ounces low fat 2% plain Greek yogurt

Lean Foods - These are foods that contain 10g to 20g total fat. When consuming these foods, there should be no serving of healthy fat. These include the following:

- **Fish:** Tuna (bluefin steak), salmon, herring, farmed catfish, and mackerel
- **Lean beef:** Ground, steak, and roast
- **Lamb:** All cuts
- **Pork:** Pork chops, pork tenderloin, and all parts. Make sure to remove the skin
- **Ground turkey and other meats:** 85% to 94% lean
- **Chicken:** Any dark meat
- **Meatless options:** 15 ounces extra-firm tofu, 3 whole eggs (up to two times per week), 4 ounces reduced-fat skim cheese, 8 ounces part-skim ricotta cheese, and 5 ounces tempeh

Healthy Fat Servings - Healthy fat servings are allowed under this diet. They should contain 5 grams of fat and less than grams of Carbs. Regardless of what type of Optavia Diet plan you follow, make sure that you add between 0 and 2 healthy fat servings daily. Below are the different healthy fat servings that you can eat:

- 1 teaspoon oil (any kind of oil)
- 1 tablespoon low carbohydrate salad dressing
- 2 tablespoons reduced-fat salad dressing
- 5 to 10 black or green olives
- 1 ½ ounce avocado
- 1/3-ounce plain nuts including peanuts, almonds, pistachios
- 1 tablespoon plain seeds such as chia, sesame, flax, and pumpkin seeds
- ½ tablespoon regular butter, mayonnaise, and margarine

The Green Foods

This section will discuss the green servings that you still need to consume while following the Optavia Diet Plan. These include all kinds of vegetables that have been categorized from lower, moderate, and high in terms of carbohydrate content. One serving of vegetables should be at ½ cup unless otherwise specified.

Lower Carbohydrate - These are vegetables that contain low amounts of Carbs. If you are following the 5&1 Optavia Diet plan, then these vegetables are good for you.

- **A cup of green leafy vegetables**such as collard greens (raw), lettuce (green leaf, iceberg, butterhead, and romaine), spinach (raw), mustard greens, spring mix, bok choy (raw), and watercress.

- **½ cup of vegetables**including cucumbers, celery, radishes, white mushroom, sprouts (mung bean, alfalfa), arugula, turnip greens, escarole, nopales, Swiss chard (raw), jalapeno, and bok choy (cooked).

Moderate Carbohydrate - These are vegetables that contain moderate amounts of Carbs. Below are the types of vegetables that can be consumed in moderation:

- **½ cup of any of the following vegetables**such as asparagus, cauliflower, fennel bulb, eggplant, portabella mushrooms, kale, cooked spinach, summer squash (zucchini and scallop).

Higher Carbs - Foods that are under this category contain a high amount of starch. Make sure to consume limited amounts of these vegetables.

- **½ cup of the following vegetables**like chayote squash, red cabbage, broccoli, cooked collard and mustard greens, green or wax beans, kohlrabi, kabocha squash, cooked leeks, any peppers, okra, raw scallion, summer squash such as straightneck and crookneck, tomatoes, spaghetti squash, turnips, jicama, cooked Swiss chard, and hearts of palm.

Foods That Are Not Allowed

There are many types of foods that are not allowed for the Optavia Diet Plan. These foods either contain high amounts of fats or Carbs that can contribute to weight gain. Below are the types of foods that are not allowed under this particular diet:

- Fried foods
- Alcohol
- Milk
- Cheese
- Fruit juice
- Soda and other sweetened beverages
- Refined grains such as pasta, white rice, and white bread

How Easy Is This Diet to Follow?

When embarking on any new diet regimen, you may experience some difficulties along the way. Below are the reasons why this diet regimen is considered as the easiest to follow among all commercial diet regimens.

- **Eating out can be challenging but still possible:**If you love eating out, you can download Optavia's dining out guide. The guide comes with tips on how to navigate buffets, order beverages, and choose condiments. Aside from following the guide, you can also ask the chef to make substitutions for the ingredients used in cooking your food. For instance, you can ask the chef to serve no more than 7 ounces of steak and serve it with steamed broccoli instead of baked potatoes.

- **Opt for lean and green foods that have high fullness index:**Eat foods that contain high protein and fiber content as they can keep you full for longer periods. In fact, many nutrition experts highlight the importance of satiety when it comes to weight loss.

- **You have access to knowledgeable coaches:**If you follow the Optavia Diet plan, you have access to knowledgeable coaches and become a part of a community that will give you access to support calls and community events. You also have a standby nutrition support team that can answer your questions.

Optavia Diet Plans FAQs

You may have some questions about the Optavia Diet Plan. Below are some of the common FAQs that people ask about this diet regimen.

Which program is right for me?
Optavia offers a wide variety of programs that are designed to improve health and well-being. Choosing the right one is easy as these diet plans are designed for different individuals and their needs. However, if you are still not sure about which diet plan to follow, you can always get in touch with an Optavia coach to learn about the many options that you have.

Is it okay for me to skip fuelings?
Fuelings is very important as it is specifically formulated with the right balance of macronutrients (Carbs, fats, and protein). Proper fueling can help promote an efficient fat-burning state so that people lose fat without losing their energy. If you skip fueling, you might miss out on these important nutrients including your daily dose of vitamins and minerals. Now, if you accidentally skip your fuelings within 24 hours, it is crucial to double up so that you don't miss the nutrition provided by your fuelings.

Which plan is best for my level of fitness?
Exercise can lead to lifelong transformation. This is the reason why specific Optavia Diet plan is designed for people who have different activity levels. Active adults who engage in 45 minutes of light to moderate exercise can benefit from the 5&1 Plan. Always talk with your coach on which plan is great for your age and activity level.

Can I rearrange my fuelings especially if I work on long days or night duty?
Yes. You can rearrange the timing of your fuelings depending on your schedule. What is important is that you consume your fuelings and lean and green meals within 24 hours. So, whether you work at night or on regular hours, make sure that you eat your meals every 2 or 3 hours throughout the time that you are awake.

How often should I eat my meals?
The Optavia Diet plan teaches you the habit of eating healthy. You are encouraged to eat six small meals daily. As mentioned earlier, you are encouraged to eat every two to three hours from your waking time. Thus, start your day with fuelings and eat your lean and green meals in between your fuelings. It is recommended that you eat your first meal within an hour of waking to ensure optimal blood sugar. This is also a good strategy for hunger control.

LEAN & GREEN RECIPES

1-Pesto Zucchini Noodles

Time: 30 minutes   **Serve:** 4

Ingredients:

- 4 zucchini, spiralized
- 1 tbsp avocado oil
- 2 garlic cloves, chopped
- 2/3 cup olive oil
- 1/3 cup parmesan cheese, grated
- 2 cups fresh basil
- 1/3 cup almonds
- 1/8 tsp black pepper
- ¾ tsp sea salt

Directions:

1. Add zucchini noodles into a colander and sprinkle with ¼ teaspoon of salt. Cover and let sit for 30 minutes. Drain zucchini noodles well and pat dry.
2. Preheat the oven to 400 F.
3. Place almonds on a parchment-lined baking sheet and bake for 6-8 minutes.
4. Transfer toasted almonds into the food processor and process until coarse.
5. Add olive oil, cheese, basil, garlic, pepper, and remaining salt in a food processor with almonds and process until pesto texture.
6. Heat avocado oil in a large pan over medium-high heat.
7. Add zucchini noodles and cook for 4-5 minutes.
8. Pour pesto over zucchini noodles, mix well and cook for 1 minute.
9. Serve immediately with baked salmon.

Nutritional Value (Amount per Serving):

Calories 525   Fat 47.4 g   Carbs 9.3 g   Sugar 3.8 g   Protein 16.6 g   Cholesterol 30 mg

2-Baked Cod & Vegetables

Time: 30 minutes   **Serve:** 4

Ingredients:

- 1 lb cod fillets
- 8 oz asparagus, chopped
- 3 cups broccoli, chopped
- ¼ cup parsley, minced
- ½ tsp lemon pepper seasoning
- ½ tsp paprika
- ¼ cup olive oil
- ¼ cup lemon juice
- 1 tsp salt

Directions:

1. Preheat the oven to 400 F. Line baking sheet with parchment paper and set aside.
2. In a small bowl, mix together lemon juice, paprika, olive oil, lemon pepper seasoning, and salt.
3. Place fish fillets in the middle of the parchment paper. Place broccoli and asparagus around the fish fillets.
4. Pour lemon juice mixture over the fish fillets and top with parsley.
5. Bake in preheated oven for 13-15 minutes.
6. Serve and enjoy.

Nutritional Value (Amount per Serving):

Calories 240   Fat 14.1 g   Carbs 7.6 g   Sugar 2.6 g   Protein 23.7 g   Cholesterol 56 mg

3-Parmesan Zucchini

Time: 30 minutes   **Serve:** 4

Ingredients:

- 4 zucchini, quartered lengthwise
- 2 tbsp fresh parsley, chopped
- 2 tbsp olive oil
- ¼ tsp garlic powder
- ½ tsp dried basil
- ½ tsp dried oregano
- ½ tsp dried thyme
- ½ cup parmesan cheese, grated
- Pepper
- Salt

Directions:

1. Preheat the oven to 350 F. Line baking sheet with parchment paper and set aside.
2. In a small bowl, mix together parmesan cheese, garlic powder, basil, oregano, thyme, pepper, and salt.
3. Arrange zucchini onto the prepared baking sheet and drizzle with oil and sprinkle with parmesan cheese mixture.
4. Bake in preheated oven for 15 minutes then broil for 2 minutes or until lightly golden brown.
5. Garnish with parsley and serve immediately.

Nutritional Value (Amount per Serving):

Calories 244   Fat 16.4 g   Carbs 7 g   Sugar 3.5 g   Protein 14.5 g   Cholesterol 30 mg

4-Chicken Zucchini Noodles

Time: 25 minutes   **Serve:** 2

Ingredients:

- 1 large zucchini, spiralized
- 1 chicken breast, skinless & boneless
- ½ tbsp jalapeno, minced
- 2 garlic cloves, minced
- ½ tsp ginger, minced
- ½ tbsp fish sauce
- 2 tbsp coconut cream
- ½ tbsp honey
- ½ lime juice
- 1 tbsp peanut butter
- 1 carrot, chopped
- 2 tbsp cashews, chopped
- ¼ cup fresh cilantro, chopped
- 1 tbsp olive oil
- Pepper
- Salt

Directions:

1. Heat olive oil in a pan over medium-high heat.
2. Season chicken breast with pepper and salt. Once the oil is hot then add chicken breast into the pan and cook for 3-4 minutes per side or until cooked.
3. Remove chicken breast from pan. Shred chicken breast with a fork and set aside.
4. In a small bowl, mix together peanut butter, jalapeno, garlic, ginger, fish sauce, coconut cream, honey, and lime juice. Set aside.
5. In a large mixing bowl, combine together spiralized zucchini, carrots, cashews, cilantro, and shredded chicken.
6. Pour peanut butter mixture over zucchini noodles and toss to combine.
7. Serve immediately and enjoy.

Nutritional Value (Amount per Serving):

Calories 353   Fat 21.1 g   Carbs 20.5 g   Sugar 10.8 g   Protein 24.5 g   Cholesterol 54 mg

5-Tomato Cucumber Avocado Salad

Time: 15 minutes   **Serve:** 4

Ingredients:

- 12 oz cherry tomatoes, cut in half
- 5 small cucumbers, chopped
- 3 small avocados, chopped
- ½ tsp ground black pepper
- 2 tbsp olive oil
- 2 tbsp fresh lemon juice
- ¼ cup fresh cilantro, chopped
- 1 tsp sea salt

Directions:

1. Add cherry tomatoes, cucumbers, avocados, and cilantro into the large mixing bowl and mix well.
2. Mix together olive oil, lemon juice, black pepper, and salt and pour over salad.
3. Toss well and serve immediately.

Nutritional Value (Amount per Serving):

Calories 442   Fat 37.1 g   Carbs 30.3 g   Sugar 9.4 g   Protein 6.2 g   Cholesterol 0 mg

6-Creamy Cauliflower Soup

Time: 30 minutes   **Serve:** 6

Ingredients:

- 5 cups cauliflower rice
- 8 oz cheddar cheese, grated
- 2 cups unsweetened almond milk
- 2 cups vegetable stock
- 2 tbsp water
- 1 small onion, chopped
- 2 garlic cloves, minced
- 1 tbsp olive oil
- Pepper
- Salt

Directions:

1. Heat olive oil in a large stockpot over medium heat.
2. Add onion and garlic and cook for 1-2 minutes.
3. Add cauliflower rice and water. Cover and cook for 5-7 minutes.
4. Now add vegetable stock and almond milk and stir well. Bring to boil.
5. Turn heat to low and simmer for 5 minutes.
6. Turn off the heat. Slowly add cheddar cheese and stir until smooth.
7. Season soup with pepper and salt.
8. Stir well and serve hot.

Nutritional Value (Amount per Serving):

Calories 214   Fat 16.5 g   Carbs 7.3 g   Sugar 3 g   Protein 11.6 g   Cholesterol 40 mg

7-Taco Zucchini Boats

Time: 70 minutes   **Serve:** 4

Ingredients:

- 4 medium zucchinis, cut in half lengthwise
- ¼ cup fresh cilantro, chopped
- ½ cup cheddar cheese, shredded
- ¼ cup water
- 4 oz tomato sauce
- 2 tbsp bell pepper, mined
- ½ small onion, minced
- ½ tsp oregano
- 1 tsp paprika
- 1 tsp chili powder
- 1 tsp cumin
- 1 tsp garlic powder
- 1 lb lean ground turkey
- ½ cup salsa
- 1 tsp kosher salt

Directions:

1. Preheat the oven to 400 F. Add ¼ cup of salsa in the bottom of the baking dish.
2. Using a spoon hollow out the center of the zucchini halves.
3. Chop the scooped-out flesh of zucchini and set aside ¾ of a cup chopped flesh.
4. Add zucchini halves in the boiling water and cook for 1 minute. Remove zucchini halves from water.
5. Add ground turkey in a large pan and cook until meat is no longer pink. Add spices and mix well.
6. Add reserved zucchini flesh, water, tomato sauce, bell pepper, and onion. Stir well and cover, simmer over low heat for 20 minutes.
7. Stuff zucchini boats with taco meat and top each with one tablespoon of shredded cheddar cheese.
8. Place zucchini boats in baking dish. Cover dish with foil and bake in preheated oven for 35 minutes.
9. Top with remaining salsa and chopped cilantro. Serve and enjoy.

Nutritional Value (Amount per Serving):

Calories 297   Fat 13.7 g   Carbs 17.2 g   Sugar 9.3 g   Protein 30.2 g   Cholesterol 96 mg

8-Healthy Broccoli Salad

Time: 25 minutes   **Serve:** 6

Ingredients:

- 3 cups broccoli, chopped
- 1 tbsp apple cider vinegar
- ½ cup Greek yogurt
- 2 tbsp sunflower seeds
- 3 bacon slices, cooked and chopped
- 1/3 cup onion, sliced
- ¼ tsp stevia

Directions:

1. In a mixing bowl, mix together broccoli, onion, and bacon.
2. In a small bowl, mix together yogurt, vinegar, and stevia and pour over broccoli mixture. Stir to combine.
3. Sprinkle sunflower seeds on top of the salad.
4. Store salad in the refrigerator for 30 minutes.
5. Serve and enjoy.

Nutritional Value (Amount per Serving):

Calories 90   Fat 4.9 g   Carbs 5.4 g   Sugar 2.5 g   Protein 6.2 g   Cholesterol 12 mg

9-Delicious Zucchini Quiche

Time: 60 minutes   **Serve:** 8

Ingredients:

- 6 eggs
- 2 medium zucchini, shredded
- ½ tsp dried basil
- 2 garlic cloves, minced
- 1 tbsp dry onion, minced
- 2 tbsp parmesan cheese, grated
- 2 tbsp fresh parsley, chopped
- ½ cup olive oil
- 1 cup cheddar cheese, shredded
- ¼ cup coconut flour
- ¾ cup almond flour
- ½ tsp salt

Directions:

1. Preheat the oven to 350 F. Grease 9-inch pie dish and set aside.
2. Squeeze out excess liquid from zucchini.
3. Add all ingredients into the large bowl and mix until well combined. Pour into the prepared pie dish.
4. Bake in preheated oven for 45-60 minutes or until set.
5. Remove from the oven and let it cool completely.
6. Slice and serve.

Nutritional Value (Amount per Serving):

Calories 288   Fat 26.3 g   Carbs 5 g   Sugar 1.6 g   Protein 11 g   Cholesterol 139 mg

10-Turkey Spinach Egg Muffins

Time: 30 minutes   **Serve:** 3

Ingredients:

- 5 egg whites
- 2 eggs
- ¼ cup cheddar cheese, shredded
- ¼ cup spinach, chopped
- ¼ cup milk
- 3 lean breakfast turkey sausage
- Pepper
- Salt

Directions:

1. Preheat the oven to 350 F. Grease muffin tray cups and set aside.
2. In a pan, brown the turkey sausage links over medium-high heat until sausage is brown from all the sides.
3. Cut sausage in ½-inch pieces and set aside.
4. In a large bowl, whisk together eggs, egg whites, milk, pepper, and salt. Stir in spinach.
5. Pour egg mixture into the prepared muffin tray.
6. Divide sausage and cheese evenly between each muffin cup.
7. Bake in preheated oven for 20 minutes or until muffins are set.
8. Serve warm and enjoy.

Nutritional Value (Amount per Serving):

Calories 123   Fat 6.8 g   Carbs 1.9 g   Sugar 1.6 g   Protein 13.3 g   Cholesterol 123 mg

11-Chicken Casserole

Time: 40 minutes   **Serve:** 4

Ingredients:

- 1 lb cooked chicken, shredded
- ¼ cup Greek yogurt
- 1 cup cheddar cheese, shredded
- ½ cup salsa
- 4 oz cream cheese, softened
- 4 cups cauliflower florets
- 1/8 tsp black pepper
- ½ tsp kosher salt

Directions:

1. Add cauliflower florets into the microwave-safe dish and cook for 10 minutes or until tender.
2. Add cream cheese and microwave for 30 seconds more. Stir well.
3. Add chicken, yogurt, cheddar cheese, salsa, pepper, and salt and stir everything well.
4. Preheat the oven to 375 F.
5. Bake in preheated oven for 20 minutes.
6. Serve hot and enjoy.

Nutritional Value (Amount per Serving):

Calories 429   Fat 23 g   Carbs 9.6 g   Sugar 4.7 g   Protein 45.4 g   Cholesterol 149 mg

12-Shrimp Cucumber Salad

Time: 20 minutes **Serve:** 4

Ingredients:

- 1 lb shrimp, cooked
- 1 bell pepper, sliced
- 2 green onions, sliced
- ½ cup fresh cilantro, chopped
- 2 cucumbers, sliced
- For dressing:
- 2 tbsp fresh mint leaves, chopped
- 1 tsp sesame seeds
- ½ tsp red pepper flakes
- 1 tbsp olive oil
- ¼ cup rice wine vinegar
- ¼ cup lime juice
- 1 Serrano chili pepper, minced
- 3 garlic cloves, minced
- ½ tsp salt

Directions:

1. In a small bowl, whisk together all dressing ingredients and set aside.
2. In a mixing bowl, mix together shrimp, bell pepper, green onion, cilantro, and cucumbers.
3. Pour dressing over salad and toss well.
4. Serve and enjoy.

Nutritional Value (Amount per Serving):

Calories 219 Fat 6.1 g Carbs 11.3 g Sugar 4.2 g Protein 27.7 g Cholesterol 239 mg

13-Asparagus & Shrimp Stir Fry

Time: 20 minutes   **Serve:** 4

Ingredients:

- 1 lb asparagus
- 1 lb shrimp
- 2 tbsp lemon juice
- 1 tbsp soy sauce
- 1 tsp ginger, minced
- 1 garlic clove, minced
- 1 tsp red pepper flakes
- ¼ cup olive oil
- Pepper
- Salt

Directions:

1. Heat 2 tablespoons of oil in a large pan over medium-high heat.
2. Add shrimp to the pan and season with red pepper flakes, pepper, and salt and cook for 5 minutes.
3. Remove shrimp from pan and set aside.
4. Add remaining oil in the same pan. Add garlic, ginger, and asparagus and stir frequently and cook until asparagus is tender about 5 minutes.
5. Return shrimp to the pan. Add lemon juice and soy sauce and stir until well combined.
6. Serve hot and enjoy.

Nutritional Value (Amount per Serving):

Calories 274   Fat 14.8 g   Carbs 7.4 g   Sugar 2.4 g   Protein 28.8 g   Cholesterol 239 mg

14-Turkey Burgers

Time: 30 minutes   **Serve:** 4

Ingredients:

- 1 lb lean ground turkey
- 2 green onions, sliced
- ¼ cup basil leaves, shredded
- 2 garlic cloves, minced
- 2 medium zucchini, shredded and squeeze out all the liquid
- ½ tsp black pepper
- ½ tsp sea salt

Directions:

1. Heat grill to medium heat.
2. Add all ingredients into the mixing bowl and mix until well combined.
3. Make four equal shapes of patties from the mixture.
4. Spray one piece of foil with cooking spray.
5. Place prepared patties on the foil and grill for 10 minutes. Turn patties to the other side and grill for 10 minutes more.
6. Serve and enjoy.

Nutritional Value (Amount per Serving):

Calories 183   Fat 8.3 g   Carbs 4.5 g   Sugar 1.9 g   Protein 23.8 g   Cholesterol 81 mg

15-Broccoli Kale Salmon Burgers

Time: 30 minutes   **Serve:** 5

Ingredients:

- 2 eggs
- ½ cup onion, chopped
- ½ cup broccoli, chopped
- ½ cup kale, chopped
- ½ tsp garlic powder
- 2 tbsp lemon juice
- ½ cup almond flour
- 15 oz can salmon, drained and bones removed
- ½ tsp salt

Directions:

1. Line one plate with parchment paper and set aside.
2. Add all ingredients into the large bowl and mix until well combined.
3. Make five equal shapes of patties from mixture and place on a prepared plate.
4. Place plate in the refrigerator for 30 minutes.
5. Spray a large pan with cooking spray and heat over medium heat.
6. Once the pan is hot then add patties and cook for 5-7 minutes per side.
7. Serve and enjoy.

Nutritional Value (Amount per Serving):

Calories 221   Fat 12.6 g   Carbs 5.2 g   Sugar 1.4 g   Protein 22.1 g   Cholesterol 112 mg

16-Pan Seared Cod

Time: 25 minutes   **Serve:** 4

Ingredients:

- 1 ¾ lbs cod fillets
- 1 tbsp ranch seasoning
- 4 tsp olive oil

Directions:

1. Heat oil in a large pan over medium-high heat.
2. Season fish fillets with ranch seasoning.
3. Once the oil is hot then place fish fillets in a pan and cook for 6-8 minutes on each side.
4. Serve immediately and enjoy.

Nutritional Value (Amount per Serving):

Calories 207   Fat 6.4 g   Carbs 0 g   Sugar 0 g   Protein 35.4 g   Cholesterol 97 mg

17-Quick Lemon Pepper Salmon

Time: 18 minutes   **Serve:** 4

Ingredients:

- 1 ½ lbs salmon fillets
- ½ tsp ground black pepper
- 1 tsp dried oregano
- 2 garlic cloves, minced
- ¼ cup olive oil
- 1 lemon juice
- 1 tsp sea salt

Directions:

1. In a large bowl, mix together lemon juice, olive oil, garlic, oregano, black pepper, and salt.
2. Add fish fillets in bowl and coat well with marinade and place in the refrigerator for 15 minutes.
3. Preheat the grill.
4. Brush grill grates with oil.
5. Place marinated salmon fillets on hot grill and cook for 4 minutes then turn salmon fillets to the other side and cook for 4 minutes more.
6. Serve and enjoy.

Nutritional Value (Amount per Serving):

Calories 340   Fat 23.3 g   Carbs 1.2 g   Sugar 0.3 g   Protein 33.3 g   Cholesterol 75 mg

18-Healthy Salmon Salad

Time: 20 minutes   **Serve:** 2

Ingredients:

- 2 salmon fillets
- 2 tbsp olive oil
- ¼ cup onion, chopped
- 1 cucumber, peeled and sliced
- 1 avocado, diced
- 2 tomatoes, chopped
- 4 cups baby spinach
- Pepper
- Salt

Directions:

1. Heat oil in a pan over medium-high heat.
2. Season salmon fillets with pepper and salt. Place fish fillets in a pan and cook for 4-5 minutes.
3. Turn fish fillets and cook for 2-3 minutes more.
4. Divide remaining ingredients evenly between two bowls, then top with cooked fish fillet.
5. Serve and enjoy.

Nutritional Value (Amount per Serving):

Calories 350   Fat 23.2 g   Carbs 15.3 g   Sugar 6.6 g   Protein 25 g   Cholesterol 18 mg

19-Pan Seared Tilapia

Time: 18 minutes   **Serve:** 2

Ingredients:

- 18 oz tilapia fillets
- ¼ tsp lemon pepper
- ½ tsp parsley flakes
- ¼ tsp garlic powder
- 1 tsp Cajun seasoning
- ½ tsp dried oregano
- 2 tbsp olive oil

Directions:

1. Heat olive oil in a pan over medium heat.
2. Season fish fillets with lemon pepper, parsley flakes, garlic powder, Cajun seasoning, and oregano.
3. Place fish fillets in the pan and cook for 3-4 minutes on each side.
4. Serve and enjoy.

Nutritional Value (Amount per Serving):

Calories 333   Fat 16.4 g   Carbs 0.7 g   Sugar 0.1 g   Protein 47.6 g   Cholesterol 124 mg

20-Creamy Broccoli Soup

Time: 35 minutes   **Serve:** 8

Ingredients:

- 20 oz frozen broccoli, thawed and chopped
- ¼ tsp nutmeg
- 4 cups vegetable broth
- 1 potato, peeled and chopped
- 2 garlic cloves, peeled and chopped
- 1 large onion, chopped
- 1 tbsp olive oil
- Pepper
- Salt

Directions:

1. Heat oil in a large saucepan over medium heat.
2. Add garlic and onion and sauté until onion is tender.
3. Add potato, broccoli, and broth and bring to boil. Turn heat to low and simmer for 15 minutes or until vegetables are tender.
4. Using blender puree the soup until smooth. Season soup with nutmeg, pepper, and salt.
5. Serve and enjoy.

Nutritional Value (Amount per Serving):

Calories 84   Fat 2.7 g   Carbs 10.9 g   Sugar 2.6 g   Protein 5.1 g   Cholesterol 0 mg

21-Tuna Muffins

Time: 35 minutes   **Serve:** 8

Ingredients:

- 2 eggs, lightly beaten
- 1 can tuna, flaked
- 1 tsp cayenne pepper
- 1/4 cup mayonnaise
- 1 celery stalk, chopped
- 1 1/2 cups cheddar cheese, shredded
- 1/4 cup sour cream
- Pepper
- Salt

Directions:

1. Preheat the oven to 350 F. Grease muffin tin and set aside.
2. Add all ingredients into the large bowl and mix until well combined and pour into the prepared muffin tin.
3. Bake for 25 minutes.
4. Serve and enjoy.

Nutritional Value (Amount per Serving):

Calories 185   Fat 14 g   Carbs 2.6 g   Sugar 0.7 g   Protein 13 g   Cholesterol 75 mg

22-Chicken Cauliflower Rice

Time: 25 minutes   **Serve:** 4

Ingredients:

- 1 cauliflower head, chopped
- 2 cups cooked chicken, shredded
- 1 tsp olive oil
- 1 tsp garlic powder
- 1 tsp chili powder
- 1 tsp cumin
- 1/4 cup tomatoes, diced
- Salt

Directions:

1. Add cauliflower into the food processor and process until get rice size pieces.
2. Heat oil in a pan over high heat.
3. Add cauliflower rice and chicken in a pan and cook for 5-7 minutes.
4. Add garlic powder, chili powder, cumin, tomatoes, and salt. Stir well and cook for 7-10 minutes more.
5. Serve and enjoy.

Nutritional Value (Amount per Serving):

Calories 140   Fat 3.6 g   Carbs 5 g   Sugar 2 g   Protein 22 g   Cholesterol 54 mg

23-Easy Spinach Muffins

Time: 25 minutes   **Serve:** 12

Ingredients:

- 10 eggs
- 2 cups spinach, chopped
- 1/4 tsp garlic powder
- 1/4 tsp onion powder
- 1/2 tsp dried basil
- 1 1/2 cups parmesan cheese, grated
- Salt

Directions:

1. Preheat the oven to 400 F. Grease muffin tin and set aside.
2. In a large bowl, whisk eggs with basil, garlic powder, onion powder, and salt.
3. Add cheese and spinach and stir well.
4. Pour egg mixture into the prepared muffin tin and bake 15 minutes.
5. Serve and enjoy.

Nutritional Value (Amount per Serving):

Calories 110   Fat 7 g   Carbs 1 g   Sugar 0.3 g   Protein 9 g   Cholesterol 165 mg

24-Healthy Cauliflower Grits

Time: 2 hours 10 minutes   **Serve:** 8

Ingredients:

- 6 cups cauliflower rice
- 1/4 tsp garlic powder
- 1 cup cream cheese
- 1/2 cup vegetable stock
- 1/4 tsp onion powder
- 1/2 tsp pepper
- 1 tsp salt

Directions:

1. Add all ingredients into the slow cooker and stir well combine.
2. Cover and cook on low for 2 hours.
3. Stir and serve.

Nutritional Value (Amount per Serving):

Calories 126   Fat 10 g   Carbs 5 g   Sugar 2 g   Protein 4 g   Cholesterol 31 mg

25-Spinach Tomato Frittata

Time: 30 minutes   **Serve:** 8

Ingredients:

- 12 eggs
- 2 cups baby spinach, shredded
- 1/4 cup sun-dried tomatoes, sliced
- 1/2 tsp dried basil
- 1/4 cup parmesan cheese, grated
- Pepper
- Salt

Directions:

1. Preheat the oven to 425 F. Grease oven-safe pan and set aside.
2. In a large bowl, whisk eggs with pepper and salt. Add remaining ingredients and stir to combine.
3. Pour egg mixture into the prepared pan and bake for 20 minutes.
4. Slice and serve.

Nutritional Value (Amount per Serving):

Calories 116   Fat 7 g   Carbs 1 g   Sugar 1 g   Protein 10 g   Cholesterol 250 mg

26-Tofu Scramble

Time: 17 minutes   **Serve:** 2

Ingredients:

- 1/2 block firm tofu, crumbled
- 1 cup spinach
- 1/4 cup zucchini, chopped
- 1 tbsp olive oil
- 1 tomato, chopped
- 1/4 tsp ground cumin
- 1 tbsp turmeric
- 1 tbsp coriander, chopped
- 1 tbsp chives, chopped
- Pepper
- Salt

Directions:

1. Heat oil in a pan over medium heat.
2. Add tomato, zucchini, and spinach and sauté for 2 minutes.
3. Add tofu, turmeric, cumin, pepper, and salt, and sauté for 5 minutes.
4. Garnish with chives and coriander.
5. Serve and enjoy.

Nutritional Value (Amount per Serving):

Calories 102   Fat 8 g   Carbs 5 g   Sugar 2 g   Protein 3 g   Cholesterol 0 mg

27-Shrimp & Zucchini

Time: 30 minutes   **Serve:** 4

Ingredients:

- 1 lb shrimp, peeled and deveined
- 1 zucchini, chopped
- 1 summer squash, chopped
- 2 tbsp olive oil
- 1/2 small onion, chopped
- 1/2 tsp paprika
- 1/2 tsp garlic powder
- 1/2 tsp onion powder
- Pepper
- Salt

Directions:

1. In a bowl, mix together paprika, garlic powder, onion powder, pepper, and salt. Add shrimp and toss well.
2. Heat 1 tablespoon of oil in a pan over medium heat,
3. Add shrimp and cook for 2 minutes on each side or until shrimp turns to pink.
4. Transfer shrimp on a plate.
5. Add remaining oil in a pan.
6. Add onion, summer squash, and zucchini and cook for 6-8 minutes or until vegetables are softened.
7. Return shrimp to the pan and cook for 1 minute.
8. Serve and enjoy.

Nutritional Value (Amount per Serving):

Calories 215   Fat 9 g   Carbs 6 g   Sugar 2 g   Protein 27 g   Cholesterol 239 mg

28-Baked Dijon Salmon

Time: 30 minutes   **Serve:** 5

Ingredients:

- 1 1/2 lbs salmon
- 1/4 cup Dijon mustard
- 1/4 cup fresh parsley, chopped
- 1 tbsp garlic, chopped
- 1 tbsp olive oil
- 1 tbsp fresh lemon juice
- Pepper
- Salt

Directions:

1. Preheat the oven to 375 F. Line baking sheet with parchment paper.
2. Arrange salmon fillets on a prepared baking sheet.
3. In a small bowl, mix together garlic, oil, lemon juice, Dijon mustard, parsley, pepper, and salt.
4. Brush salmon top with garlic mixture.
5. Bake for 18-20 minutes.
6. Serve and enjoy.

Nutritional Value (Amount per Serving):

Calories 217   Fat 11 g   Carbs 2 g   Sugar 0.2 g   Protein 27 g   Cholesterol 60 mg

29-Cauliflower Spinach Rice

Time: 15 minutes   **Serve:** 4

Ingredients:

- 5 oz baby spinach
- 4 cups cauliflower rice
- 1 tsp garlic, minced
- 3 tbsp olive oil
- 1 fresh lime juice
- 1/4 cup vegetable broth
- 1/4 tsp chili powder
- Pepper
- Salt

Directions:

1. Heat olive oil in a pan over medium heat.
2. Add garlic and sauté for 30 seconds. Add cauliflower rice, chili powder, pepper, and salt and cook for 2 minutes.
3. Add broth and lime juice and stir well.
4. Add spinach and stir until spinach is wilted.
5. Serve and enjoy.

Nutritional Value (Amount per Serving):

Calories 147   Fat 11 g   Carbs 9 g   Sugar 4 g   Protein 5 g   Cholesterol 23 mg

30-Cauliflower Broccoli Mash

Time: 22 minutes   **Serve:** 3

Ingredients:

- 1 lb cauliflower, cut into florets
- 2 cups broccoli, chopped
- 1 tsp garlic, minced
- 1 tsp dried rosemary
- 1/4 cup olive oil
- Salt

Directions:

1. Add broccoli and cauliflower into the instant pot.
2. Pour enough water into the instant pot to cover broccoli and cauliflower.
3. Seal pot and cook on high pressure for 12 minutes.
4. Once done, allow to release pressure naturally. Remove lid.
5. Drain broccoli and cauliflower and clean the instant pot.
6. Add oil into the instant pot and set the pot on sauté mode.
7. Add broccoli, cauliflower, rosemary, garlic, and salt and cook for 10 minutes.
8. Mash the broccoli and cauliflower mixture using a masher until smooth.
9. Serve and enjoy.

Nutritional Value (Amount per Serving):

Calories 205   Fat 17 g   Carbs 12 g   Sugar 5 g   Protein 5 g   Cholesterol 0 mg

31-Italian Chicken Soup

Time: 35 minutes   **Serve:** 6

Ingredients:

- 1 lb chicken breasts, boneless and cut into chunks
- 1 1/2 cups salsa
- 1 tsp Italian seasoning
- 2 tbsp fresh parsley, chopped
- 3 cups chicken stock
- 8 oz cream cheese
- Pepper
- Salt

Directions:

1. Add all ingredients except cream cheese and parsley into the instant pot and stir well.
2. Seal pot and cook on high pressure for 25 minutes.
3. Release pressure using quick release. Remove lid.
4. Remove chicken from pot and shred using a fork.
5. Return shredded chicken to the instant pot.
6. Add cream cheese and stir well and cook on sauté mode until cheese is melted.
7. Serve and enjoy.

Nutritional Value (Amount per Serving):

Calories 300   Fat 19 g   Carbs 5 g   Sugar 2 g   Protein 26 g   Cholesterol 109 mg

32-Tasty Tomatoes Soup

Time: 15 minutes   **Serve:** 2

Ingredients:

- 14 oz can fire-roasted tomatoes
- 1/2 tsp dried basil
- 1/2 cup heavy cream
- 1/2 cup parmesan cheese, grated
- 1 cup cheddar cheese, grated
- 1 1/2 cups vegetable stock
- 1/4 cup zucchini, grated
- 1/2 tsp dried oregano
- Pepper
- Salt

Directions:

1. Add tomatoes, stock, zucchini, oregano, basil, pepper, and salt into the instant pot and stir well.
2. Seal pot and cook on high pressure for 5 minutes.
3. Release pressure using quick release. Remove lid.
4. Set pot on sauté mode. Add heavy cream, parmesan cheese, and cheddar cheese and stir well and cook until cheese is melted.
5. Serve and enjoy.

Nutritional Value (Amount per Serving):

Calories 460   Fat 35 g   Carbs 13 g   Sugar 6 g   Protein 24 g   Cholesterol 117 mg

33-Cauliflower Spinach Soup

Time: 20 minutes   **Serve:** 2

Ingredients:

- 3 cups spinach, chopped
- 1 cup cauliflower, chopped
- 2 tbsp olive oil
- 3 cups vegetable broth
- 1/2 cup heavy cream
- 1 tsp garlic powder
- Pepper
- Salt

Directions:

1. Add all ingredients except cream into the instant pot and stir well.
2. Seal pot and cook on high pressure for 10 minutes.
3. Release pressure using quick release. Remove lid.
4. Stir in cream and blend soup using a blender until smooth.
5. Serve and enjoy.

Nutritional Value (Amount per Serving):

Calories 310   Fat 27 g   Carbs 7 g   Sugar 3 g   Protein 10 g   Cholesterol 41 mg

34-Delicious Chicken Salad

Time: 15 minutes   **Serve:** 4

Ingredients:

- 1 1/2 cups chicken breast, skinless, boneless, and cooked
- 2 tbsp onion, diced
- 1/4 cup olives, diced
- 1/4 cup roasted red peppers, diced
- 1/4 cup cucumbers, diced
- 1/4 cup celery, diced
- 1/4 cup feta cheese, crumbled
- 1/2 tsp onion powder
- 1/2 tbsp fresh lemon juice
- 1 tbsp fresh parsley, chopped
- 1 tbsp fresh dill, chopped
- 2 1/2 tbsp mayonnaise
- 1/4 cup Greek yogurt
- 1/4 tsp pepper
- 1/2 tsp salt

Directions:

1. In a bowl, mix together yogurt, onion powder, lemon juice, parsley, dill, mayonnaise, pepper, and salt.
2. Add chicken, onion, olives, red peppers, cucumbers, and feta cheese and stir well.
3. Serve and enjoy.

Nutritional Value (Amount per Serving):

Calories 172   Fat 7.9 g   Carbs 6.7 g   Sugar 3.1 g   Protein 18.1 g   Cholesterol 52 mg

35-Baked Pesto Salmon

Time: 30 minutes   **Serve:** 5

Ingredients:

- 1 3/4 lbs salmon fillet
- 1/3 cup basil pesto
- 1/4 cup sun-dried tomatoes, drained
- 1/4 cup olives, pitted and chopped
- 1 tbsp fresh dill, chopped
- 1/4 cup capers
- 1/3 cup artichoke hearts
- 1 tsp paprika
- 1/4 tsp salt

Directions:

1. Preheat the oven to 400 F. Line baking sheet with parchment paper.
2. Arrange salmon fillet on a prepared baking sheet and season with paprika and salt.
3. Add remaining ingredients on top of salmon and spread evenly.
4. Bake for 20 minutes.
5. Serve and enjoy.

Nutritional Value (Amount per Serving):

Calories 228   Fat 10.7 g   Carbs 2.7 g   Sugar 0.3 g   Protein 31.6 g   Cholesterol 70 mg

36-Easy Shrimp Salad

Time: 15 minutes   **Serve:** 6

Ingredients:

- 2 lbs shrimp, cooked
- 1/4 cup onion, minced
- 1/4 cup fresh dill, chopped
- 1/3 cup fresh chives, chopped
- 1/2 cup fresh celery, chopped
- 1/4 tsp cayenne pepper
- 1 tbsp fresh lemon juice
- 1 tbsp olive oil
- 1/4 cup mayonnaise
- 1/4 tsp pepper
- 1/4 tsp salt

Directions:

1. In a large bowl, add all ingredients except shrimp and mix well.
2. Add shrimp and toss well.
3. Serve and enjoy.

Nutritional Value (Amount per Serving):

Calories 248   Fat 8.3 g   Carbs 6.7 g   Sugar 1.1 g   Protein 35.2 g   Cholesterol 321 mg

37-Simple Haddock Salad

Time: 15 minutes   **Serve:** 6

Ingredients:

- 1 lb haddock, cooked
- 1 tbsp green onion, chopped
- 1 tbsp olive oil
- 1 tsp garlic, minced
- Pepper
- Salt

Directions:

1. Cut cooked haddock into the bite-size pieces and place on a plate.
2. Drizzle with oil and season with pepper and salt.
3. Sprinkle garlic and green onion over haddock.
4. Serve and enjoy.

Nutritional Value (Amount per Serving):

Calories 106   Fat 3 g   Carbs 0.2 g   Sugar 0 g   Protein 18.4 g   Cholesterol 56 mg

38-Baked White Fish Fillet

Time: 40 minutes   **Serve:** 1

Ingredients:

- 8 oz frozen white fish fillet
- 1 tbsp roasted red bell pepper, diced
- 1/2 tsp Italian seasoning
- 1 tbsp fresh parsley, chopped
- 1 1/2 tbsp olive oil
- 1 tbsp lemon juice

Directions:

1. Preheat the oven to 400 F. Line baking sheet with foil.
2. Place a fish fillet on a baking sheet.
3. Drizzle oil and lemon juice over fish. Season with Italian seasoning.
4. Top with roasted bell pepper and parsley and bake for 30 minutes.
5. Serve and enjoy.

Nutritional Value (Amount per Serving):

Calories 383   Fat 22.5 g   Carbs 0.8 g   Sugar 0.6 g   Protein 46.5 g   Cholesterol 2 mg

39-Air Fry Salmon

Time: 25 minutes   **Serve:** 4

Ingredients:

- 1 lbs salmon, cut into 4 pieces
- 1 tbsp olive oil
- 1/2 tbsp dried rosemary
- 1/4 tsp dried basil
- 1 tbsp dried chives
- Pepper
- Salt

Directions:

1. Place salmon pieces skin side down into the air fryer basket.
2. In a small bowl, mix together olive oil, basil, chives, and rosemary.
3. Brush salmon with oil mixture and air fry at 400 F for 15 minutes.
4. Serve and enjoy.

Nutritional Value (Amount per Serving):

Calories 182   Fat 10.6 g   Carbs 0.3 g   Sugar 0 g   Protein 22 g   Cholesterol 50 mg

40-Baked Salmon Patties

Time: 30 minutes   **Serve:** 4

Ingredients:

- 2 eggs, lightly beaten
- 14 oz can salmon, drained and flaked with a fork
- 1 tbsp garlic, minced
- 1/4 cup almond flour
- 1/2 cup fresh parsley, chopped
- 1 tsp Dijon mustard
- 1/4 tsp pepper
- 1/2 tsp kosher salt

Directions:

1. Preheat the oven to 400 F. Line a baking sheet with parchment paper and set aside.
2. Add all ingredients into the bowl and mix until well combined.
3. Make small patties from mixture and place on a prepared baking sheet.
4. Bake patties for 10 minutes.
5. Turn patties and bake for 10 minutes more.
6. Serve and enjoy.

Nutritional Value (Amount per Serving):

Calories 216   Fat 11.8 g   Carbs 3 g   Sugar 0.5 g   Protein 24.3 g   Cholesterol 136 mg

FUELING RECIPES

41-Chocolate Bars

Time: 20 minutes   **Serve:** 16

Ingredients:

- 15 oz cream cheese, softened
- 15 oz unsweetened dark chocolate
- 1 tsp vanilla
- 10 drops liquid stevia

Directions:

1. Grease 8-inch square dish and set aside.
2. Melt chocolate in a saucepan over low heat.
3. Add stevia and vanilla and stir well.
4. Remove pan from heat and set aside.
5. Add cream cheese into the blender and blend until smooth.
6. Add melted chocolate mixture into the cream cheese and blend until just combined.
7. Transfer mixture into the prepared dish and spread evenly and place in the refrigerator until firm.
8. Slice and serve.

Nutritional Value (Amount per Serving):

Calories 230   Fat 24 g   Carbs 7.5 g   Sugar 0.1 g   Protein 6 g   Cholesterol 29 mg

42-Blueberry Muffins

Time: 35 minutes   **Serve:** 12

Ingredients:

- 2 eggs
- 1/2 cup fresh blueberries
- 1 cup heavy cream
- 2 cups almond flour
- 1/4 tsp lemon zest
- 1/2 tsp lemon extract
- 1 tsp baking powder
- 5 drops stevia
- 1/4 cup butter, melted

Directions:

1. Preheat the oven to 350 F. Line muffin tin with cupcake liners and set aside.
2. Add eggs into the bowl and whisk until mix.
3. Add remaining ingredients and mix to combine.
4. Pour mixture into the prepared muffin tin and bake for 25 minutes.
5. Serve and enjoy.

Nutritional Value (Amount per Serving):

Calories 190   Fat 17 g   Carbs 5 g   Sugar 1 g   Protein 5 g   Cholesterol 55 mg

43-Chia Pudding

Time: 20 minutes   **Serve:** 2

Ingredients:

- 4 tbsp chia seeds
- 1 cup unsweetened coconut milk
- 1/2 cup raspberries

Directions:

1. Add raspberry and coconut milk into a blender and blend until smooth.
2. Pour mixture into the glass jar.
3. Add chia seeds in a jar and stir well.
4. Seal the jar with a lid and shake well and place in the refrigerator for 3 hours.
5. Serve chilled and enjoy.

Nutritional Value (Amount per Serving):

Calories 360   Fat 33 g   Carbs 13 g   Sugar 5 g   Protein 6 g   Cholesterol 0 mg

44-Avocado Pudding

Time: 20 minutes   **Serve:** 8

Ingredients:

- 2 ripe avocados, peeled, pitted and cut into pieces
- 1 tbsp fresh lime juice
- 14 oz can coconut milk
- 2 tsp liquid stevia
- 2 tsp vanilla

Directions:

1. Add all ingredients into the blender and blend until smooth.
2. Serve immediately and enjoy.

Nutritional Value (Amount per Serving):

Calories 317   Fat 30 g   Carbs 9 g   Sugar 0.5 g   Protein 3 g   Cholesterol 0 mg

45-Peanut Butter Coconut Popsicle

Time: 15 minutes   **Serve:** 12

Ingredients:

- 1/2 cup peanut butter
- 1 tsp liquid stevia
- 2 cans unsweetened coconut milk

Directions:

1. Add all ingredients into the blender and blend until smooth.
2. Pour mixture into the Popsicle molds and place in the freezer for 4 hours or until set.
3. Serve and enjoy.

Nutritional Value (Amount per Serving):

Calories 155   Fat 15 g   Carbs 4 g   Sugar 2 g   Protein 3 g   Cholesterol 0 mg

46-Delicious Brownie Bites

Time: 20 minutes   **Serve:** 13

Ingredients:

- 1/4 cup unsweetened chocolate chips
- 1/4 cup unsweetened cocoa powder
- 1 cup pecans, chopped
- 1/2 cup almond butter
- 1/2 tsp vanilla
- 1/4 cup monk fruit sweetener
- 1/8 tsp pink salt

Directions:

1. Add pecans, sweetener, vanilla, almond butter, cocoa powder, and salt into the food processor and process until well combined.
2. Transfer brownie mixture into the large bowl. Add chocolate chips and fold well.
3. Make small round shape balls from brownie mixture and place onto a baking tray.
4. Place in the freezer for 20 minutes.
5. Serve and enjoy.

Nutritional Value (Amount per Serving):

Calories 108   Fat 9 g   Carbs 4 g   Sugar 1 g   Protein 2 g   Cholesterol 0 mg

47-Pumpkin Balls

Time: 15 minutes   **Serve:** 18

Ingredients:

- 1 cup almond butter
- 5 drops liquid stevia
- 2 tbsp coconut flour
- 2 tbsp pumpkin puree
- 1 tsp pumpkin pie spice

Directions:

1. In a large bowl, mix together pumpkin puree and almond butter until well combined.
2. Add liquid stevia, pumpkin pie spice, and coconut flour and mix well.
3. Make small balls from mixture and place onto a baking tray.
4. Place in the freezer for 1 hour.
5. Serve and enjoy.

Nutritional Value (Amount per Serving):

Calories 96   Fat 8 g   Carbs 4 g   Sugar 1 g   Protein 2 g   Cholesterol 0 mg

48-Smooth Peanut Butter Cream

Time: 10 minutes   **Serve:** 8

Ingredients:

- 1/4 cup peanut butter
- 4 overripe bananas, chopped
- 1/3 cup cocoa powder
- 1/4 tsp vanilla extract
- 1/8 tsp salt

Directions:

1. Add all ingredients into the blender and blend until smooth.
2. Serve immediately and enjoy.

Nutritional Value (Amount per Serving):

Calories 101   Fat 5 g   Carbs 14 g   Sugar 7 g   Protein 3 g   Cholesterol 0 mg

49-Vanilla Avocado Popsicles

Time: 20 minutes   **Serve:** 6

Ingredients:

- 2 avocadoes
- 1 tsp vanilla
- 1 cup almond milk
- 1 tsp liquid stevia
- 1/2 cup unsweetened cocoa powder

Directions:

1. Add all ingredients into the blender and blend until smooth.
2. Pour blended mixture into the Popsicle molds and place in the freezer until set.
3. Serve and enjoy.

Nutritional Value (Amount per Serving):

Calories 130   Fat 12 g   Carbs 7 g   Sugar 1 g   Protein 3 g   Cholesterol 0 mg

50-Chocolate Popsicle

Time: 20 minutes   **Serve:** 6

Ingredients:

- 4 oz unsweetened chocolate, chopped
- 6 drops liquid stevia
- 1 1/2 cups heavy cream

Directions:

1. Add heavy cream into the microwave-safe bowl and microwave until just begins the boiling.
2. Add chocolate into the heavy cream and set aside for 5 minutes.
3. Add liquid stevia into the heavy cream mixture and stir until chocolate is melted.
4. Pour mixture into the Popsicle molds and place in freezer for 4 hours or until set.
5. Serve and enjoy.

Nutritional Value (Amount per Serving):

Calories 198   Fat 21 g   Carbs 6 g   Sugar 0.2 g   Protein 3 g   Cholesterol 41 mg

51-Raspberry Ice Cream

Time: 10 minutes   **Serve:** 2

Ingredients:

- 1 cup frozen raspberries
- 1/2 cup heavy cream
- 1/8 tsp stevia powder

Directions:

1. Add all ingredients into the blender and blend until smooth.
2. Serve immediately and enjoy.

Nutritional Value (Amount per Serving):

Calories 144   Fat 11 g   Carbs 10 g   Sugar 4 g   Protein 2 g   Cholesterol 41 mg

52-Chocolate Frosty

Time: 20 minutes   **Serve:** 4

Ingredients:

- 2 tbsp unsweetened cocoa powder
- 1 cup heavy whipping cream
- 1 tbsp almond butter
- 5 drops liquid stevia
- 1 tsp vanilla

Directions:

1. Add cream into the medium bowl and beat using the hand mixer for 5 minutes.
2. Add remaining ingredients and blend until thick cream form.
3. Pour in serving bowls and place them in the freezer for 30 minutes.
4. Serve and enjoy.

Nutritional Value (Amount per Serving):

Calories 137   Fat 13 g   Carbs 3 g   Sugar 0.5 g   Protein 2 g   Cholesterol 41 mg

53-Chocolate Almond Butter Brownie

Time: 26 minutes   **Serve:** 4

Ingredients:

- 1 cup bananas, overripe
- 1/2 cup almond butter, melted
- 1 scoop protein powder
- 2 tbsp unsweetened cocoa powder

Directions:

1. Preheat the air fryer to 325 F. Grease air fryer baking pan and set aside.
2. Add all ingredients into the blender and blend until smooth.
3. Pour batter into the prepared pan and place in the air fryer basket and cook for 16 minutes.
4. Serve and enjoy.

Nutritional Value (Amount per Serving):

Calories 82   Fat 2 g   Carbs 11 g   Sugar 5 g   Protein 7 g   Cholesterol 16 mg

54-Peanut Butter Fudge

Time: 20 minutes   **Serve:** 20

Ingredients:

- 1/4 cup almonds, toasted and chopped
- 12 oz smooth peanut butter
- 15 drops liquid stevia
- 3 tbsp coconut oil
- 4 tbsp coconut cream
- Pinch of salt

Directions:

1. Line baking tray with parchment paper.
2. Melt coconut oil in a saucepan over low heat. Add peanut butter, coconut cream, stevia, and salt in a saucepan. Stir well.
3. Pour fudge mixture into the prepared baking tray and sprinkle chopped almonds on top.
4. Place the tray in the refrigerator for 1 hour or until set.
5. Slice and serve.

Nutritional Value (Amount per Serving):

Calories 131   Fat 12 g   Carbs 4 g   Sugar 2 g   Protein 5 g   Cholesterol 0 mg

55-Almond Butter Fudge

Time: 10 minutes   **Serve:** 18

Ingredients:

- 3/4 cup creamy almond butter
- 1 1/2 cups unsweetened chocolate chips

Directions:

1. Line 8*4-inch pan with parchment paper and set aside.
2. Add chocolate chips and almond butter into the double boiler and cook over medium heat until the chocolate-butter mixture is melted. Stir well.
3. Pour mixture into the prepared pan and place in the freezer until set.
4. Slice and serve.

Nutritional Value (Amount per Serving):

Calories 197   Fat 16 g   Carbs 7 g   Sugar 1 g   Protein 4 g   Cholesterol 0 mg

56-Mocha Mousse

Time: 20 minutes   **Serve:** 8

Ingredients:

- 1/2 cup coffee strong brewed, cooled
- 2 cups heavy whipping cream
- 6 oz unsweetened chocolate, chopped
- 1 tsp coffee extract

Directions:

1. In a large bowl, whip heavy cream and set aside.
2. Melt chocolate in a microwave-safe bowl.
3. Add coffee and coffee extract in melted chocolate and stir well.
4. Pour chocolate mixture into the whipped cream and stir until just combined.
5. Place in refrigerator for 30 minutes.
6. Serve and enjoy.

Nutritional Value (Amount per Serving):

Calories 211   Fat 22 g   Carbs 7 g   Sugar 0.2 g   Protein 3 g   Cholesterol 41 mg

57-Pumpkin Mousse

Time: 20 minutes   **Serve:** 12

Ingredients:

- 2 tsp pumpkin pie spice
- 1 tsp liquid stevia
- 2 cups heavy cream
- 15 oz can pumpkin puree
- 15 oz cream cheese
- 1 tsp vanilla
- Pinch of salt

Directions:

1. In a large bowl, blend together pumpkin and cream cheese until smooth.
2. Add remaining ingredients and beat until fluffy.
3. Pipe into the serving glasses and place in the refrigerator for 1 hour.
4. Serve and enjoy.

Nutritional Value (Amount per Serving):

Calories 209   Fat 19 g   Carbs 5 g   Sugar 1 g   Protein 3 g   Cholesterol 66 mg

58-Chocolate Mousse

Time: 10 minutes   **Serve:** 4

Ingredients:

- 1/2 cup unsweetened cocoa powder
- 1 1/4 cup heavy cream
- 5 drop stevia
- 4 oz cream cheese
- 1/2 tsp vanilla

Directions:

1. Add all ingredients to the blender and blend until smooth and.
2. Pipe mixture into the serving glasses and place them in the refrigerator for 1 hour.
3. Serve chilled and enjoy.

Nutritional Value (Amount per Serving):

Calories 254   Fat 25 g   Carbs 7 g   Sugar 0.4 g   Protein 5 g   Cholesterol 83 mg

59-Pound Cake

Time: 65 minutes   **Serve:** 10

Ingredients:

- 4 eggs
- 1/4 cup cream cheese
- 1/4 cup butter
- 1 tsp baking powder
- 1 tbsp coconut flour
- 1 cup almond flour
- 1/2 cup sour cream
- 1 tsp vanilla
- 1 cup monk fruit sweetener

Directions:

1. Preheat the oven to 350 F. Grease 9-inch cake pan and set aside.
2. In a large bowl, mix together almond flour, baking powder, and coconut flour.
3. In a separate bowl, add cream cheese and butter and microwave for 30 seconds. Stir well and microwave for 30 seconds more.
4. Stir in sour cream, vanilla, and sweetener. Stir well.
5. Pour cream cheese mixture into the almond flour mixture and stir until just combined.
6. Add eggs in batter one by one and stir until well combined.
7. Pour batter into the prepared cake pan and bake for 55 minutes.
8. Remove cake from the oven and let it cool completely.
9. Slice and serve.

Nutritional Value (Amount per Serving):

Calories 211   Fat 17 g   Carbs 8 g   Sugar 5 g   Protein 3 g   Cholesterol 89 mg

60-Almond Butter Cookies

Time: 28 minutes   **Serve:** 7

Ingredients:

- 6 oz almond butter
- 1/3 cup pumpkin puree
- 1/4 tsp pumpkin pie spice
- 1 tsp liquid stevia

Directions:

1. Preheat the oven to 350 F. Line baking sheet with parchment paper and set aside.
2. Add all ingredients into the food processor and process until just combined.
3. Drop spoonfuls of mixture onto the prepared baking sheet.
4. Bake for 18 minutes.
5. Let the cookies cool completely.
6. Serve and enjoy.

Nutritional Value (Amount per Serving):

Calories 88   Fat 7 g   Carbs 3 g   Sugar 1 g   Protein 3 g   Cholesterol 0 mg